You Bet Your Life!

The
Top 10 Reasons
You Need a
Professional
Patient Advocate
by Your Side

Get the Healthcare
You Need and Deserve

by

Trisha Torrey

Every Patient's Advocate

You Bet Your Life!
The Top 10 Reasons You Need a Professional Patient Advocate by Your Side

© 2015 by Trisha Torrey, Every Patient's Advocate

Discounts for bulk-orders of this book are available by contacting the author. She is also available for speaking engagements to groups of patients or professionals.

Published by

diagKNOWsis Media
PO Box 53
Baldwinsville, NY 13027
1-888-478-6588

YouBetYourLifeBooks.com
YBYL@diagKNOWsis.com

The information in this book is not intended to substitute for medical or legal advice. It is intended only to help patients and their loved ones navigate the complex and dysfunctional health care system. Should you require medical care, you are advised to consult the professionals who can provide that care. Should you require legal advice, please contact an attorney to help you.

ISBN— 978-0-9828014-7-5

Printed in the United States of America

Dedication

It's not easy being a pioneer in a new
profession, one that didn't exist less than
a decade ago.

I count among my blessings the hundreds of
pioneering, private, professional, patient
advocates who are the members of the
Alliance of Professional Health Advocates.
I have the privilege of working with them
every day.

This book is dedicated to "my advocates,"
and their hard work in building a system that
helps patients get the care they need, at the
time they need it, at a cost they can afford.

Trisha Torrey

Every Patient's Advocate
July 2015

Table of Contents

Find direct links to the resources in this book at:

www.YouBetYourLifeBooks.com/10Reasons/Resources

Introduction

Medical Nirvana Is Now Extinct

D o you long, as I do, for the Marcus Welby days?

If you're missing that reference, Marcus Welby, MD, was the kindly TV doctor of the 1970s, played by Robert Young, who was always successful, and always cared. Each week, in the span of one hour, he solved the most difficult of patient situations, was always there for his patients; physically, mentally and emotionally.

And then... those patients never received a bill for his services.

Medical nirvana! And today, impossible to find, no matter where in the world you live.

Fast forward to today and you'll find the healthcare system has become almost unrecognizable. Why does the doctor spend so little time with you? Why won't your doctors talk to each other? Why do they send you for so many tests; do you really need them all? And why is it that you're paying so much more than you used to for things insurance used to cover?

Those questions, and many more, remain unanswered, or if they are answered, you don't like what you hear.

I don't blame you!

It's a dangerous potion: less care and more cost. Frustration and confusion. Too much of the wrong information, and not enough that is understandable. Mistakes made, and you don't know it, and you can't fix them.

How are you supposed to get what you need, when you need it, at a price you can afford?

Enter patient advocates. Specifically professional, independent, patient advocates; people who improve the quality of your life, perhaps extend the quantity of your life... The people you must have by your side if you are diagnosed with, or being treated for, any sort of condition or disease that is more than an annoying sniffle or a bumped head.

A Scary Diagnosis Is Like Getting Thrown Into Jail

You're driving home from an evening out when flashing red lights come up behind you. You pull your car over, as required, are asked for your license and registration, and the next thing you know you've been arrested and thrown into jail.

Whaaat? Why? Having never been in jail before, you have no idea what to expect. You're floored, flustered and fearful. They're talking charges and lawyers and one phone call, and you're in your head trying to sort out why you were pulled over in the first place. You hadn't had a drink for more than two hours, you weren't speeding - so - what? You don't understand the words they are using, except that you will be there at least overnight. Your car is still parked on the side of the road. Your spouse is expecting you home but won't have any idea where you are...

Your life has been turned upside down, totally without warning, and you are now being handled by people who don't speak your language (they speak legal, you speak people), may not respect you, want to tell you what decisions to make, and hold your fate in their hands.

Yes, they hold YOUR fate in THEIR hands.

In a parallel life:

You're standing in your front yard, watering your garden, greeting neighbors as they walk by, and you notice a golf ball sized lump on your torso. Seems odd, so you phone your doctor who also thinks it's odd. The next thing you know, you've had surgery to remove the lump and have been diagnosed with a terminal form of cancer, told you have just a few months to live.

Whaaat? Why? Having never had anything worse than pneumonia before, you have no idea what to expect. You're floored, flustered and fearful. They're talking surgery and chemo, and you're still in your head trying to sort out how you could have landed there from watering your garden!

You don't understand the words they are using, except that you must make a decision in a hurry because it is, after all, your life.

Now your life has been turned upside down, totally without warning, and you are being handled by people who don't speak your language (they speak medical, you speak people), may not respect you, want to tell you what decisions to make, and hold your fate in their hands. Not only that, it will cost you your life savings to figure it all out.

Yes, they hold YOUR fate in THEIR hands.

Déjà vu, right?

The first story is made up. The second story happened to me.[1]

In the first story, the only logical next step is to call a lawyer, or call your spouse or partner who will then call a lawyer. You have been forced into a situation that is non-comprehensible to you and you need a professional to help - literally - bail you out. There is no way you can handle such a situation without true expertise, and the true experts are lawyers.

The police seem to be the ones who have caused your untenable situation. A lawyer will be the one to help figure out why you were arrested, what will happen next, and what it will take to get you bailed out and the charges dropped, if possible.

So who do you call in the second story?

After all, it's the doctors who have put you in this untenable situation. Typically you might think it's another doctor who would solve it for you - but I'm here to tell you that it's far more complicated than that. It's one reason I wrote this book

In fact, in my own story (which took place in 2004), it turned out the doctors and pathologists were wrong. I had no cancer. I had no malignancy at all. And I had no one around to help me figure it out. Only out of desperation, luck, and the seat of my pants was I able to figure out I was not terminally ill. In more than a decade since, I've never had any form of treatment for that misdiagnosis. I don't even have a real name for a correct diagnosis.

---

1 http://everypatientsadvocate.com/who-is-trisha/misdiagnosis

And, yes, unfortunately, it cost me most of my life savings to get it straightened out, even though I had health insurance.

Enter Patient Advocates

Oh how I wished I had access to a professional who could have navigated me through those treacherous medical care waters! You'll find additional parts of my story peppered throughout this book to illustrate the gravity of each reason you need a patient advocate by your side when you face similar treacherous waters.

My approach in 2004 was way too DIY[2] and could have cost me my health and my life. There was no professional patient advocate for me to call. Today there is no question in my mind that if I had been able to consult with a professional advocate, I never would have been taken to the brink of chemo and radiation, and I would not have lost my savings.

Just what exactly can a professional patient advocate do to help you that you can't do for yourself?

Plenty.

To try to navigate the healthcare system on your own when faced with a difficult diagnosis or decisions to make, is foolhardy. Just like you would never try to represent yourself in court, or perform surgery on yourself, or weather an audit from the IRS on your own, (heck, I won't even cut my own hair!) you should not try to tackle your journey through medical care on your own either - for at least the 10 reasons outlined in this book.

We'll get to those 10 reasons shortly, but before we do, let's look at exactly who these professional patient advocates are and how their work can benefit you.

At the very least, professional advocates are a solution. At the most, they are angels.

Find direct links to the resources in this book at:

www.YouBetYourLifeBooks.com/10Reasons/Resources

---

2 DIY = Do It Yourself

Chapter One

What Is a Professional Patient Advocate?

The description "patient advocate" is very generic, describing anyone who steps up to help a patient.

Someone who helps another human being who is sick or debilitated is, in effect, that patient's advocate. That might be you or your spouse, your friend, neighbor or co-worker, or a doctor or nurse or other medical personnel. You/they are all advocates when you help someone else improve their problematic health situation.

Further, there might be a variety of helpful tasks any advocate performs: From driving someone to doctor appointments, to making sure they take their prescription drug at the right time in the right dose, to helping someone research a new diagnosis, or make a treatment decision. Or, they may sit by a patient's bedside in the hospital, reconcile their medical bills, or even help them choose the right insurance plan.

I expect you will look at that list of tasks and think, "I can do those things!" And so, yes, you probably can do most of them.

But - what happens when you don't know the right questions to ask? What happens when you sit in on a doctor's appointment but you don't understand what the doctor said any better than your partner did? Or, what if you do all that great web research about a new treatment, only to find out later that you relied on a pharmaceutical company's recommendations for a loved one, and the treatment or cure ended up costing thousands of dollars more than it needed to? Or that the best treatment for the disease that's killing your child is turned down by your insurance, and you don't know how to get past that denial?

THOSE are the things professional advocates know how to do. Just like you have no idea how to put up bail to get out of jail, nonprofessionals don't know the potholes or pitfalls of getting through the medical system either. It's too easy for patients to fall through the cracks no matter how well-meaning their friends and family advocates are.

Intentional Obfuscation[3]

I'm sure you'll agree that during the past ten years or so, the medical system has become much more complicated to maneuver. It's more difficult than ever to get what we need, or at least what we think we need.

There are several reasons for this, all of which bolster the argument that we need professional patient advocates, so let's take a look at them.

Begin by following the money. All the healthcare moneymakers - doctors, hospitals, insurers, pharmaceutical companies, medical device companies, large pharmacies and pharmacy management companies - are working harder than ever to suck every possible dollar from the system - US. They are sucking the money from us both as patients and taxpayers.

At the same time the moneymakers are trying to make as much money as possible, insurers are also working diligently to be sure they don't spend one more dime than they are required to. They make their money by saving money - not spending it even in the places they promise to spend it. Doctors are writing prescriptions and prescribing treatments that are more expensive than ever before, and insurers are denying coverage more frequently than ever before.

More and more of the costs are being shouldered by us patient-taxpayers than ever before.

As a result, patients have begun to think more like consumers, and for the first time in history are demanding more accountability for what they are getting for their money and their efforts. But, unlike hot dogs or sausage, the system requires intentional cover-up to make it palatable. As patients demand more, the moneymakers are hunkering down to reduce transparency, like a shell game - a shell game of life and death.

---

3 (There it is. I always wanted to use the word "obfuscation" in a book I wrote. Check that one off the list! To obfuscate means to confuse or make something unclear.)

And so it follows, that as the system continues to become more opaque, and therefore more difficult to navigate, and more expensive, there is just no possible way that patients can get the best from the system on their own without professional help. Two of the most important aspects of our lives are our health and our money. Aren't they worth the turn to professional help?

What Advocacy Help Is Available?

There are dozens of ways professional advocates can help you or your loved one improve your outcomes while you journey through the healthcare system. In fact, there is a master list of these services that is updated regularly.[4] Let's look at some of the highlights. Advocates may:

- accompany you to medical appointments or stay by your bedside in the hospital

- help you learn more about your medical condition and treatment options

- help you make difficult medical decisions

- help you maintain a healthy pregnancy and raise healthy babies

- teach you pain management techniques

- help you navigate the insurance maze

- help you file health insurance claims, dispute denials, and manage or reduce your hospital and medical bills

- help your family come to agreement on decisions that need to be made for a loved one who needs health-related assistance

- find legal assistance after a medical error

- track paperwork and records

- help you file for social security disability or other assistance

- .. or help with many additional services, too.

I could list dozens more aspects of healthcare that an advocate can help you with, but they really boil down to two general titles—care and cost.

---

4 http://AdvoConnection.com/advocacy-services/

Care
Help with anything that regards your actual medical condition, treatment, the people and facilities that provide care, available medical research, drugs and devices and more.

Cost
If you live in the United States then you have learned, more vehemently in the past few years than ever before, that there is no care without a cost consideration. Cost considerations range from paying for your health insurance, to all the associated out-of-pocket costs like premiums, co-pays, co-insurance and more. The moneymakers WILL take their piece of the ever-increasing pie.

Advocates Come in Many Flavors

Not all advocates can help you with all services. Sometimes that's because they haven't been trained or don't have experience in one aspect of advocacy. For example, a medical billing specialist might not be the best person to sit by a patient's bedside in the hospital.

Patient advocates go by a variety of names. In some cases what they choose to call themselves depends on a job title, or the work they do. In other cases they choose what they will be called based on personal preference. Here are some of the monikers you might see, all of whom are advocates:

- Patient advocate (or health advocate)
- Patient navigator (or health navigator)
- Consumer health advocate
- Care and case manager or coordinator
- Care and case partner
- Care and case advocate
- Ombudsman
- Eldercare professional
- Family mediator
- Health coach
- Health insurance advisors or disability advisor
- Medical bill reviewer or claims reviewer
- And many more.

For purposes of this book, we will use the title "patient advocate" to represent all these titles and others that may be found in use by the general public.

Like the services they provide, most advocates focus on either care or the cost of care in the work they can do for patients.

The Allegiance Factor

More important than what an advocate is called and just as important as the work she does for you, is a concept that speaks to the nexus of efficacy and conflicts of interest. It's what we advocates call The Allegiance Factor.

The Allegiance Factor refers to the source of your advocate, or more to the point, the source of the advocate's paycheck. The person or entity paying your advocate has everything to do with how objective, and possibly thorough and effective, an advocate's advice may be, as follows:

- When an advocate draws her paycheck from a hospital, her allegiance is to the hospital. Hospital advocates, who may also be called patient representatives, patient experience professionals, ombudsmen and other names, usually work for the risk management department of the hospital. As such, their jobs are focused on keeping the hospital out of hot water.

  A hospital advocate MAY be able to help the patient (or maybe not.) Her job is to keep lawsuits at bay and save the hospital money – which she does by helping patients, but only to the extent it doesn't interfere with the hospital's needs and her job requirements.

  This is also true for hospital navigators who operate differently from hospital advocates, yes, but who are just as beholden to their employer. This is a relatively new concept in hospitals—navigators—and they are often assigned to cancer patients. While having one by your side can be very reassuring, and these navigators can help with some aspects of care, they are not able to make any recommendations outside the process and treatment already prescribed. So, for example, they cannot help you change doctors, nor get a second opinion, nor can they help with transitions of care (discussed more fully in Reason #4) nor get anywhere near a review of your medical bills.

- If an advocate draws her paycheck from an insurance company, then her allegiance is to the insurance company. Insurers hire advocates to work with patients more like customer service representatives do. They teach their advocates to make recommendations that will save the insurer money. As long as their recommendations benefit both – fine. But if not, it would be difficult to picture an insurer's patient advocate making a recommendation to the patient that might be very good for the patient, but expensive for the insurer.

Could it happen? Maybe. Is it the usual course of business? No way.

On the other hand, private, independent advocates are exactly that - private and independent. You hire them directly, so they work for you, not some entity that stands to make money or lose money by working with you.

Yes, you pay directly for their help, and no, you can't be reimbursed by insurance for the work they have done for you. (We'll take a look at the cost of a private advocate in Chapter Twelve.)

This actually makes sense, and it's better for you that it works that way. Why? Because the minute the advocate's services could be paid by insurance or Medicare or any other payer, it would mean the insurer could determine what they would, or would not pay for, which means they would control the care you receive.

That's no better than the existing system where our doctors' hands are tied. The last thing we want is to tie an advocate's hands, too. The reasons you're having trouble to begin with are due to control issues. A private advocate helps shift that control to you.

What About Help From a Family Member or Friend?

I used to think there would be nothing better than having a doctor or nurse in the family to pitch in when one of us had a health challenge. To an extent that's still true (and, wonderfully and remarkably enough, my daughter-in-law is a nurse practitioner! We're so lucky!)

But I've had to temper that wish a bit. Now I think it may even be better to have a private, professional, knowledgeable patient advocate in the family.

Having a loved one who can pitch in to help out in a health crisis is a godsend, no doubt about it, because none of us - NONE OF US - can do it alone.

But for many of the reasons listed here in this book, a loved one is really only about a two on a scale of 1 to 10 for the kind of support you need if you have been diagnosed with something difficult, or face difficult or lifelong treatment. As you read and understand each reason, you'll see more and more why a family member or friend can only be so helpful, even if he or she is a nurse or a doctor.

You wouldn't ask an amateur doctor to treat you. You wouldn't ask an amateur lawyer to get you out of jail. You wouldn't ask an amateur accountant to do your taxes... and you don't want an amateur to play the role of advocate either.

Including, truthfully, most doctors and nurses, who are real amateurs when it comes to navigating the system. To prove that point: if they could help you navigate, then we wouldn't need advocates at all.

The Top 10 Reasons You Need a Private Patient Advocate by Your Side

And thus - this book. We've looked at the many titles and forms of assistance a patient advocate can supply to you.

But one thing is clear:

If you want to be sure that you'll get the highly professional assistance you need, with no conflicts-of-interest, then the best help you can get will be from an independent, private, professional patent advocate.

There are dozens of reasons, but 10 of those reasons stand out.

So let's get started.

Find direct links to the resources in this book at:

www.YouBetYourLifeBooks.com/10Reasons/Resources

Chapter Two

Reason #1

YDKWYDK
You Don't Know What You Don't Know

I t's true in every aspect of life: if you know the questions to ask, you can probably find the answer somewhere. The same is true with our journeys through medical care. From asking a doctor, to googling a word or phrase, we can find an answer.

But, what if you don't know the questions to ask?

The problem with this reason, and the reason it's first on the list, is because not knowing the questions or the answers means you may never get what you need. Whether it's a question about your medical condition, or about how much it will cost you to get it cleared up, you will fail in your quest to improve your health, or your outcomes, or the cost of either, when you don't know what you don't know.

Examples:

Hannah was bent over from pains in her lower right side. Barely able to breath, she was rushed to the emergency department of her local hospital; a hospital she knew was covered by her health insurance. The ER doctor sent her to surgery to remove her appendix. She even had the wherewithal to double check that the surgeon was covered by her insurance, and asked how long she would be there post-surgery. The surgery went well. She was able to rest easy based on the questions she had asked. Three weeks after she got home, she received a bill from an anesthesiologist expecting her to pay for his services during her surgery.

What Hannah didn't know: just because the hospital and surgeon were covered by her insurance, that didn't mean everything about her surgery and hospital stay were covered. The anesthesiologist was considered "out of network." Hannah was forced to pay almost $6,000 she had not anticipated.

Patricia was diagnosed with a rare form of lymphoma after having a small lump removed from her torso. By the time the doctor shared the diagnosis with her, two pathology labs had reviewed the sectional slides of the lump, agreeing on the terminal nature of the diagnosis. She was given a few months to live and told to begin chemo immediately to buy herself an extra year.

What Patricia didn't know: Yes - this is more of my own story. And yes, as explained in the introduction to this book, the doctors were wrong, and I was misdiagnosed. What I didn't find out until years later is the danger of being diagnosed from medical tests that require professional review during July and August.

In fact, what most of us don't know is that most labs and hospitals are staffed beginning July 1 with recent medical school graduates; young people who have just completed their medical school but have spent very little time working directly with patients, and even less time analyzing evidence in the form of medical tests. Studies show this to be more of a problem in academic medical institutions (like your local university-related hospital), although can also be a factor for any hospital that hires first-year residents (formerly called interns.)[5]

Of course, these young people just don't have the experience to accurately diagnose anything unusual, not without having more experienced personnel to help them.

But those experienced personnel are too often poolside or on the golf course, or anywhere else a well-to-do professional might take a vacation, because beginning July through the rest of the summer

---

5   http://www.amednews.com/article/20110715/profession/307159997/8/
Please note this study is from 2011. More recent studies pronounce the "July Effect" to be negligible on death rates. However, no studies, to date, have measured the number of medical errors in general during the summer (which may not have caused deaths) and logically new doctors would be very apt to make mistakes. Regardless, an advocate can be sure you have only a solidly experienced doctor helping you.

You Don't Know the Right People Either

Along with the fact that YDKWYDK is the fact that we rarely know the right people to care for us either.

I frequently have this conversation with doctors and some nurses. I ask them, "If you or a loved one experience strange symptoms and you know you need to seek care, what do you do?"

The answer every time (and I do mean every time) is, "I would call my friend who is a _____ (fill in the blank with the right specialist)."

Then I ask how long it would take to get the appointment. The response is, "She would fit me in as a professional courtesy."

We patients don't have friends who cover the spectrum of specialties - at least not those friends. Even if we do, they may not be covered by our insurance. And, unfortunately, it often takes weeks for us to get an appointment.

Further, it should go without saying, that just because a doctor shows up on our list of possibilities doesn't mean he or she is any good at what they do. This is where the Allegiance Factor plays out: insurers want you to work with the doctor who will cost them the least, not the one that might be best. Your doctor will refer you to a friend, not necessarily someone who is any good.

So - consider this an adjunct to the YDKWYDK reason. We may never know the right people before we need them, but knowing how to find them - immediately - is vital. That's what private, professional advocates do.

is vacation time, too. Like all workers, experienced doctors and pathologists take time off during the summer, especially if they have children who are out of school for the summer.

These are just two examples of YDKWYDK and how that can be detrimental to your health or your wallet. I could cite hundreds more.

Much of what we don't know relates to the money-makers.

Further, both the system and the body of medical knowledge change every day. It's impossible for any human being to keep up with it all. And, as much as we wish it weren't true, doctors are human beings just like the rest of us.

So your best bet, maybe your only chance to get the best outcome for your own situation, is to find a patient advocate who keeps up with processes, the changes in policies, the shifts in the system, the navigational knowledge, knows the resources to find the most current information, and is willing to do so for one individual - you.

A private professional advocate is the person who DOES know what you don't know. That's what she does for a living. That is, after all, why the profession exists.

Find direct links to the resources in this book at:

www.YouBetYourLifeBooks.com/10Reasons/Resources

Chapter Three

Reason #2

Your Emotions Get In the Way

When I work with private advocates to help them understand marketing, I teach them that the bulk of clients who will want to work with them can be described within (what I call) the FUDGE Theory.

See if any of these emotions sound familiar:

F = Fear
U = Uncertainty
D = Doubt
G = Guilt
E = Exhaustion

Let's look at these emotions and see how they apply to Reason #2 - and you.

• **Fear**

If you or a loved one have ever been diagnosed with something difficult or dire, you know that your world just stops - and then it begins to spin. Panic sets in. A million questions flood your brain, not the least of which regard your fears of your prognosis, and whether that means pain, agony, expensive illness, and of course your demise. Everything else in your life just falls by the wayside. You just can't deal.

NO ONE, and I mean NO ONE, is in any position to be making the best decisions for themselves at that point. Adrenaline does funny things to us and even the most intelligent people among us can't think straight when we are gripped by fear. Anxiety is never a decision-maker's friend.

Fear is also a hallmark of emotion for loving family and caregivers, too. Have you been married for decades and can't imagine living without your partner? Is the patient the breadwinner? Is someone going to ask you to pull the plug?

- **Uncertainty**

Now what? You've been diagnosed with something horrible, or you've been hurt in an accident and can't truly process what's going on (those great drugs that keep you pain free but leave you fuzzy, or even comatose.)

Everyone is in such a hurry. No one is paying attention to your questions, or they are using words you don't understand. You know the doctor wrote a prescription, but you can't remember what it was for. Will you have to take this drug for the rest of your life? Will your spouse ever walk again? Can you afford the treatment being recommended?

Is it the right diagnosis? Should you get a second opinion? That treatment sounds so painful - how can you be sure it's the right answer?

And don't forget - YDKWYDK - You don't know what you don't know!

Adding to your fears, are these layers of uncertainty, too. That is; IF you can process well enough to even be uncertain.

- **Doubt**

Second guessing, especially when it comes to medical decision-making, will be a hallmark of your journey through the system. At any given time you may doubt your providers, your insurance coverage, yourself, your decisions, and even your loved ones.

You've seen two doctors, you've gotten two different opinions, you aren't even sure one of them is right.

Your insurer denied permission for a test your doctor insists you must have. Now you're beginning to doubt whether you have the right coverage.

If you are a caregiver, you may have doubts about the choices your loved one has been making. Or you may disagree with the proposed treatment options. Or you may wish your loved one would make one choice, but he or she seems to lean toward another.

How can you know what's right? How can you know what will work? Where can you get answers?

It may be a seed of doubt, or a whole avalanche, but it is impossible to navigate medical problems without questioning almost every step.

- **Guilt**

Ohhh yes. There's nothing like a horrible medical experience to make guilt rear its ugly head.

Guilt - as in beating yourself up over questions like, Was my medical problem caused by an accident I could have prevented? Will my medical care eat through my family's entire life savings? Would I have avoided all this if I had taken better care of myself? What will happen to my family if I die? And many others, of course.

Then there is guilt that influences how decisions are made. Patients may choose a treatment option because a family member insists on it, and not because it would be their first choice. An illustration of that would be an elderly person who would prefer not to be treated for a cancer diagnosis, but goes through with chemo anyway because his wife pleads with him to do so.

There is also guilt that is less based on the current medical situation and is more about the history of the relationship. An adult child makes decisions for her parent because she feels guilty that she lives so far away, or because the last time the parent was conscious they had an argument.

It's possible your own guilty conscious has been stoked now, too.

- ## Exhaustion

Perhaps less of an emotion and more of a fact of life is the overwhelming feeling of exhaustion. Mental, physical, or emotional exhaustion can influence our decision-making in so many negative ways.

Exhaustion usually sends us down the path of least resistance instead of the path that will help us achieve our best outcomes. In my own story, I got so little sleep in the months of fear and uncertainty, that it would have been easy for me to just give in to chemo, or even to reject any sort of treatment all together, even though I had no real basis for choosing either one.

Caregivers may experience exhaustion more than anyone else in the entire patient entourage. A caregiver might be the elderly spouse, or the adult child who balances her full time job and her family, too. All that required attention leaves little time for resting and regrouping needed by the caregiver; exhaustion may become the norm.

- ## And a "bonus" emotion - Anger

(Sorry - it doesn't fit neatly with FUDGE, but it's still important!)

Remember, two of the most personal and important aspects to our lives are our health and our money. Medical problems affect both negatively, and as a result, even beyond dealing specifically with the problem at hand, it can make us angry.

We're angry that we have to deal with problems (it's never convenient to be sick or hurt, is it?), we are angry that we can't seem to get what we need. We may be angry that our insurance company has denied payment for a treatment the doctor recommends, or - and this is one of the worst - our situation may be due to a medical error - and we become angry that someone or something did that to us. (I've been there. The anger is the primary reason I now do the work I do!)

Anger can negatively affect every aspect of our health, including creating its own symptoms.

Once emotions begin to rule our heads, it becomes impossible to make the right decisions, except perhaps by luck. Our brains just don't operate the way they do when we are healthy, and without being at the top of our thinking and decision-making games, we run the risk of making decisions we will regret - and pay for - later.

While this may sound like simply a logical conclusion, it has been borne out by research, too. Since 2014, at least two medical research studies have shown this to be true.[6]

What we need is peace of mind.

Enter professional patient advocates, who are not emotionally invested, and who can neutralize all that negativity with patience, facts, and guidance.

Private patient advocates are experts at providing that peace of mind.

Your advocate will be invested in your care and outcomes, and can balance out your negative emotions - or even your wishful thinking - with a more objective reality, helping you to take your next steps and make your important decisions.

You're entitled to all the emotions you experience. So go ahead and feel them all, but let that professional advocate keep you on the even keel needed to move forward.

---

6 Invisible Risks, Emotional Choices — Mammography and Medical Decision Making (Lisa Rosenbaum, MD) published in the New England Journal of Medicine, 2014

Emotions and Health Decisions (Ferrer, Klein, Lerner, Reyna, Keltner, from the National Cancer Institute, Harvard University, Cornell University and UC Berkeley) published by Harvard University Press, 2015

Find direct links to the resources in this book at:

www.YouBetYourLifeBooks.com/10Reasons/Resources

Chapter Four

Reason #3

Your Providers Practice with
One Arm Tied Behind Their Backs

Your doctor is in a hurry. He's in a bigger hurry this year than he was last year. Next year will probably be even more difficult to get more than a few minutes of his time...

Thing is, if your doctor had a choice, he or she would probably spend unlimited time with you. Doctors keep their time with you short not because that's what they want to do; rather because that's what they must do to stay in business. This is rarely something patients think about, but it has such an effect on our care, that you need to understand it.

Here's the problem:

Over the past ten or more years, doctors have been paid less and less for the work they do. Imagine that. Imagine if you went to work, and for each hour you spent, you were paid less, year after year. Yes, it's like that. But not exactly.

Doctors get paid two ways.

First - if you have a co-pay they get money directly from you. That might be $10 or it might be $50 or more depending on your health plan and payer (insurance company, Medicare, Medicaid, etc).

Doctors also get paid for working with you through a system of reimbursements from your payer (insurance, Medicare, or another). That payment they receive is based on the things they do or sell to you. The more things your doctor does, the more she gets paid; things like examining you, prescribing for you, treating you, or testing you. When she files a report with your health plan or payer she lists all the things she did during your appointment, along with a specific code, called a CPT code, that she knows she can get paid for, and that's what her reimbursement is for meeting with you.

What don't doctors get paid for? They don't get paid for talking to you!

There is no reimbursement for a conversation or discussion. They can't get paid for explaining things to you, or answering your questions. They can't get paid for discussing different treatment options to you. They can't get paid for explaining why they have prescribed a certain drug or how often you should take it and why, what foods or beverages or activities you should avoid while taking it... in short... with no reimbursement for time, your doctor needs to spend as little time actually talking to you as possible because every minute spent with you means a minute that can't be spent with an additional patient that day - one they can do more things to and for, and get paid more for.

An additional reason you aren't getting what you need from your doctor is that reimbursements have gone down each year. But the expenses for maintaining a medical office have not. Rent goes up, employees get paid more (not to mention the cost for THEIR health insurance!), the electric bill is higher... So how can a doctor stay in business if reimbursements go down even as expenses go up?

The answer is simple, and goes to the heart of the doctor's time with you. That is....

The doctor schedules more patients in a day. The more patients he sees, the more things he can do to and for patients, the more he can get paid. That simple.

But then, there is one more logical next step. Say your doctor works a 10-hour day. Until the past few years when reimbursements began declining, she would see 20 patients in that 10 hour day which meant up to a half-hour to spend with each patient and that patient's paperwork (or electronic record keeping). But today, because reimbursements have gone so low, in order to just make as much money as she used to make then she must see 40 patients in a day, meaning only 15 minutes per patient. And, that's not 15 minutes of appointment time; that's 15 minutes of appointment and follow up record keeping which can take half or more of the time spent on a patient, even though it's not working directly with the patient.

There is one other wrinkle in this expanding time warp. The amount of time you get with your doctor can also be affected by the health insurance plan you have, or the payer you have, too. In general (although there are some exceptions) the more you (or your employer) pays for your health insurance the more time you might get because higher cost plans generally reimburse at higher rates.

If you have a government payer, like Medicare, Medicaid, Tricare, or another one, even a state payer, that may explain why you are having so much trouble finding a doctor at all, much less one that will spend any time with you.

Who Is Practicing Medicine on You?

It won't surprise you to learn that your doctor doesn't get to make the call on what path to follow for your diagnosis and treatment. You don't either.

In the process of treating you, your doctor will make recommendations that require you get permission from your insurer. It might be that you need to see a specialist, or that you need a specific test or prescription. Maybe you need something more extensive, like surgery or radiation or chemo.

In all those cases, your insurer is likely to say no. Yes, that's right. When you have lesser insurance, not only does the doctor get reimbursed less, but your coverage won't allow for many tests and procedures without a larger co-pay from you. When the doctor recommends you get a test, or when she wants to prescribe a more expensive drug, your insurer might say no. You may be told you need to pay for that test or treatment from your own pocket.

We have to ask, exactly who is practicing medicine here?

What are you supposed to do? And what will your doctor do? Your doctor's reaction may be based on whether she can make money from whatever it is she has recommended. If she is the surgeon, then she will step in to make the case on your behalf with your insurer or payer to get your surgery covered. But if she has prescribed a drug and the insurer says no, she may not do that for you. If you want that drug you'll be expected to try to get

In a Doctor's Perfect World

Most doctors are as unhappy with this reimbursement model that provides no room for conversations as we are. If left to their own devices, and if they didn't have to worry about keeping the lights on and their staffs paid, doctors would spend as much time with you as you wanted and needed.

But the reality is - most can't. It's not really even a decision they can make because there is no way for them to tilt the balance toward spending time with patients.

In any other service profession, the professional is paid based on time and results. Doctors are paid neither for time NOR results. In fact, if taken to its conspiracy-theoryesque conclusions, if the doctor doesn't do his job, doesn't make you better, then you will return, and he can do more things to you to get paid more.

Which is why you need a patient advocate by your side.

authorization on your own.

And Then There's this Problem Which Will Take You by Surprise

You may be thinking that none of these problems are your problems because you have good health insurance. You (or your employer) pay higher premiums because you think that's how you can get better care. It's worth it to you to pay extra to get what you need!

Not so fast. I'm quite sure you didn't see this one coming....

Consider:

... a middle aged woman showed up at the ER with an upset stomach and heartburn. They ran a number of tests including blood tests and a CT scan. Eventually she was given some TUMS, her symptoms were relieved, and she was sent home.... Until she got a call that the CT scan showed "something", an MRI was needed, then an endoscopy was recommended... after a series of mishaps, miscalls, and too much medicine, she ended up losing her left leg.[7]

How could this have happened?

Remember - doctors get paid by doing things: diagnosing, treating, testing, prescribing. The more diagnosing, testing,

---

7   http://www.kevinmd.com/blog/2015/06/how-heartburn-caused-a-patient-to-lose-her-left-leg.html

treating and prescribing they do, the more money they make.

As it turns out, the person with the great insurance - is a treasure trove! Chances are very good that the woman lost her leg because she had great insurance.

Yes, it's true, if you have the more extensive and expensive health plan, then you are likely to get more tests and procedures approved. That includes tests and procedures you don't really need.

You may be getting too much care.[8] It's called "overtreatment" and it's very lucrative for the moneymakers like doctors, hospitals, testing labs, pharmaceutical companies and medical device makers (all but the insurers.)

"The Waiter Will Spit In My Soup"

Many patients are afraid to ask their doctors questions, fearful that asking questions will upset the doctor, and may result in substandard care, as if the doctor won't provide what they need because they questioned whether they needed it.

I have never heard of a doctor who actually did that; but then, I'm not sure a patient would know if that had actually happened.

However, you may find you face your doctor with some fear and trepidation, too.

If so, know that a professional advocate knows how to bridge that gap -- making sure you get the answers to your questions without putting the doctor on the defensive, creating a win-win-win scenario for you, your doctor and your advocate, too.

Perhaps even more lucrative—and dangerous for patients—is "overdiagnosis."[9] You can guess what that would be; diagnosing someone beyond their real problem, then racking up the bucks for all the treatment they don't really need.

So, it's true. You may be getting tests you don't really need, or the doctor may be recommending surgery that won't really help you, or any of thousands of tests and procedures that won't necessarily improve your health or condition, but will certainly increase the moneymaker's income.

---

8 http://well.blogs.nytimes.com/2012/08/27/overtreatment-is-taking-a-harmful-toll

9 http://time.com/3379349/overdiagnosis-and-overtreatment/

How a Professional Patient Advocate Can Help

You may have no idea you aren't getting what you need from the doctor or the system - or that you are getting too much. It may never have occurred to you that you can't get your questions answered because of the system, and not because your doctor is a jerk. I'm sure you don't know when you are being over-tested because the doctor can get paid more, or you may not have realized that the reason it's so difficult to find a doctor is because most doctors preferred to be paid what they think is fair, as opposed to what patients can afford.....

Professional patient advocates know where these landmines are located. They know how to make sure you get your questions answered. They help with those transitions of care that tend to make patients fall through the cracks. They can be sure you have the information you need to decide whether surgery is the right answer - for YOU - and they can go to bat for you with the insurance company or payer if your doctor recommends something, you agree it's needed and important, and the payer says no.

Your advocate is YOUR advocate, not beholden to anyone but you. A paycheck from elsewhere won't stand in the way of you getting what is right for you.

Chapter Five

Reason #4

No One is Coordinating Your Care

We just got our arms around the way lack of time negatively affects our ability to get the care we need. Now let's add insult to injury.

Your care isn't being coordinated.

Most of us have experienced the fact that our doctors just don't communicate with each other. Your cardiologist isn't talking to your orthopedist, who isn't talking to your endocrinologist.... None of those doctors are coordinating your prescription drugs or other treatment recommendations. They are operating in silos.

Coordinating care consists of making sure records from other doctors are reviewed and conversations with other doctors take place. It consumes a great deal of time. The more complex the problem or the more comorbidities[10] you have, the more time care coordination takes, and the less likely doctors are to take that time, because just like talking to you, there is little or no reimbursement for care coordination.[11]

---

10 "Comorbidity" means two or more diseases present at the same time, like diabetes and heart disease, or allergies and high blood pressure.

11 As of January 2015, Medicare began reimbursing $42 per patient for care coordination. In a doctor's world, that's not even enough to dial the phone or send an email. There is no reimbursement for patients who are not on Medicare. http://www.medpagetoday.com/PublicHealthPolicy/Medicare/47275

Now, add time constraints to other issues, like egos, and you can see the root of this problem.

As a result, you come away from the doctor, fill your prescription or go for therapy... Yet, despite the fact that you're doing what you agreed to do, you are suffering symptoms you didn't have before, or one of the drugs isn't working the way it should, or your allergies are kicking up, or your memory seems a little fuzzy, or your sciatica is worse than ever....

Most patients have these kinds of problems and blame their own bodies. We think WE are to blame for our own problems! We think our own bodies, uniquely, aren't responding the way they should.

But, as it turns out, way too often the problems have been created by the treatment prescribed - or not prescribed - because, again, our providers aren't coordinating our care. We rarely blame the doctors who would have known better than to make the recommendations they did if they had actually talked to each other.

Further, when we have to go back to the doctor, they will probably be paid again! Being right often requires coordinating our care. So, there is no reward for them being right.

More Coordination Problems

We've already described the results of the limited-or-no time factor as it relates to the time doctors spend talking with you or coordinating your care. But this no-reimbursement-for-time extends even further, beyond your doctor.

Professionals call them "transitions of care." They are the hand-off activities where patient care can fall through the cracks, and patients don't get what they need. Some will be obvious to you, like, when a patient goes home from the hospital but doesn't understand instructions because they weren't provided, or were provided so quickly that the patient, who might be taking drugs which affect her cognition, can't remember. Others are less obvious, like making sure you get a phone call with test results - while you're thinking you didn't get the phone call because everything is OK. (It may not be.)

These transitions, when done right, can have a huge positive effect on our outcomes. But when they aren't coordinated, they can be not just problematic, but dangerous.

It's extremely rare to find anyone in the system - not the doctors, nor the hospitals - who will coordinate care transitions for us. And we can't do it ourselves when we are sick or debilitated.

Who Can We Turn to for Care Coordination?

Of course, you know the answer by now.

Private advocates to the care coordination rescue!

A private advocate can be your care coordination angel in many ways. He or she can go through your medical records with you to be sure they are correct. They can accompany you to the doctor's office to ask about potential drug conflicts, or to be sure your allergies have been taken into account before a prescription is written.

When it comes to transitions, they are the ones who make sure all the pieces fit together. They can review your many prescriptions to be sure there are no conflicts. You won't be discharged from the hospital without knowing that your new prescriptions will be available for you to take at home. You won't end up in a rehab that your insurance won't pay for. Or you won't even be sent to rehab if there is an effective alternative that can be managed from home.

They can even take care of coordinating details that aren't medical, but may have a huge influence on your ability to get well. For example, if you need to be hospitalized, they may be the ones to be sure your pets are taken care of in your absence. Or they can help coordinate information sharing among your children who live out of state but want to know what your status is.

None of us can afford for our care to go uncoordinated, and therefore cause us additional problems. That's why a private advocate, one who knows where the potential pitfalls are, and knows the right questions to ask, and resources to gather, is so crucial at these times.

Find direct links to the resources in this book at:

www.YouBetYourLifeBooks.com/10Reasons/Resources

Chapter Six

Reason #5

You Need Protection
from Medical Mistakes

H a! A medical mistake? Just like a car accident, those never happen to anyone you know... or do they?

In fact, preventable (yes - preventable!) medical errors are the #3 killer in the United States, behind only heart disease and cancer. That is 440,000 deaths each year.[12] And that's only hospital deaths.[13]

(Would we sit up and take notice if the entire population of Atlanta died accidently in one year? or Miami?)

That doesn't even count the number of deaths that result from someone who is prescribed the wrong drug, for example, or is misdiagnosed (my "favorite" mistake, of course.)

Every day you come closer to being one of those statistics. They are catching up to us all. And, sadly, when you are the victim, as I was, then the statistic is 100% of you.

---

12 A New, Evidence-based Estimate of Patient Harms Associated with Hospital Care, John T. James, PhD, Journal of Patient Safety, September 2013

13 http://www.npr.org/sections/health-shots/2013/09/20/224507654/how-many-die-from-medical-mistakes-in-u-s-hospitals

Hospital Mistakes

Preventable medical errors in hospitals were, at one time, called "never events" by the National Quality Forum. Today they are called "serious reportable events,"[14] but of course, that doesn't change the original intent - that they should never happen. Here is the NQF's list[15]:

Surgical Events
- Surgery performed on the wrong body part
- Surgery performed on the wrong patient
- Wrong surgical procedure on a patient
- Retention of a foreign object in a patient after surgery or other procedure
- Intraoperative or immediately post-operative death in a normal healthy patient

Product or Device Events
- Patient death or serious disability associated with the use of contaminated drugs, devices, or biologics provided by the healthcare facility
- Patient death or serious disability associated with the use or function of a device in patient care in which the device is used or functions other than as intended
- Patient death or serious disability associated with intravascular air embolism that occurs while being cared for in a healthcare facility

Patient Protection Events
- Infant discharged to the wrong person
- Patient death or serious disability associated with patient disappearance for more than four hours

---

14   In 2011, the healthcare lobby successfully changed the name from "never events" to "serious reportable events." That doesn't change the errors they are.

15   https://www.qualityforum.org/Topics/SREs/List_of_SREs.aspx

- Patient suicide, or attempted suicide resulting in serious disability, while being cared for in a healthcare facility

Care Management Events

- Patient death or serious disability associated with a medication error

- Patient death or serious disability associated with a hemolytic reaction due to the administration of ABO-incompatible blood or blood products (transfusion of the wrong blood type)

- Maternal death or serious disability associated with labor or delivery on a low-risk pregnancy while being cared for in a healthcare facility

- Patient death or serious disability associated with hypoglycemia, the onset of which occurs while the patient is being cared for in a healthcare facility

- Death or serious disability kernicterus associated with failure to identify and treat jaundice in newborns

- Stage 3 or 4 pressure ulcers acquired after admission to a healthcare facility

- Patient death or serious disability due to spinal manipulative therapy

Environmental Events

- Patient death or serious disability associated with an electric shock while being cared for in a healthcare facility

- Any incident in which a line designated for oxygen or other gas to be delivered to a patient contains the wrong gas or is contaminated by toxic substances

- Patient death or serious disability associated with a burn incurred from any source while being cared for in a healthcare facility

- Patient death associated with a fall while being cared for in a healthcare facility

- Patient death or serious disability associated with the use of restraints or bedrails while being cared for in a healthcare facility

Criminal Events

- Any instance of care ordered by or provided by someone impersonating a physician, nurse, pharmacist, or other licensed healthcare provider

- Abduction of a patient of any age

- Sexual assault on a patient within or on the grounds of a healthcare facility

- Death or significant injury of a patient or staff member resulting from a physical assault (i.e., battery) that occurs within or on the grounds of a healthcare facility

Savvy readers will notice one horrible medical outcome is missing from this list: **hospital acquired infections** (HAIs). The CDC estimates that 1.7 million Americans acquire these infections each year, and 99,000 die of them.[16]

Why HAIs don't appear on this list, I don't know - but they are perhaps the most frequent of the preventable harms that can come to a patient while hospitalized. If doctors, nurses and other hospital providers would simply wash and sanitize their hands, those people would not get sick and die, at least not from an HAI.

So that's hospitals. Now let's look at what's going on outside the hospital.

Misdiagnosis

You can imagine that I've focused on the error of misdiagnosis a great deal since my own odyssey in 2004. What I've learned will make your toenails curl.

Misdiagnosis is actually a number of different things. A missed diagnosis is just that - no one catches the medical problem and no treatment is given. Sometimes the patient is diagnosed with something, but it's the wrong diagnosis, and then of course, the wrong treatment ensues. Or, a third form, that the patient is

---

16 http://www.healthline.com/health-news/aging-healthcare-acquired-infections-kill-nearly-a-hundred-thousand-a-year-072713

diagnosed with a problem that doesn't really exist at all.[17] This
happens frequently to women who are told their medical problem
is "all in their heads."

The quoted rates of misdiagnosis range from 10% to 40%.[18] There
are a few different ways to look at that:

- Up to 4 out of 10 diagnoses are wrong.
- If you have 10 friends who have been diagnosed, up to 4 of
  them got the wrong diagnosis.
- If you have been to the doctor 10 times with 10 medical
  problems, they gave you the wrong diagnosis up to 4 times.

How can you know if you have been misdiagnosed?

You can't--unless and until you are willing to put a lot of effort into
research and second (and third, fourth or fifth) opinions. This is
where doctors love to tell you that medicine is an art, not a
science. As if that's an excuse.

What is clear is that you need an objective overseer to the process,
someone who is knowledgeable about the medical system, knows
what to ask and (just as importantly) HOW to ask the right
questions without creating a rift in the relationship. (This is one of
those places we are afraid the waiter-doctor might spit in our
soup.)

Yes, a patient advocate can be that person.

Mistakes at Home

In the last chapter, we took a look at care coordination which
causes many problems all by itself. In fact, one of the medical
errors we need to account for is the lack of coordination which can
result in harm. Sometimes that care coordination is a problem of
the system's making. Sometimes it's our own, even when we think
we are doing everything right.

Mistakes are made every day, innocently, because the patient
doesn't have the capability or capacity to take care of his or health
without help.

---

17 This was my case. I was diagnosed with lymphoma, but in fact, did not have
lymphoma. No alternative diagnosis has ever been determined or offered.

18   From the AHRQ: http://www.ahrq.gov/downloads/pub/advances/vol2/Schiff.pdf

- An older woman is suffering some memory problems. Her cognition is declining, as noticed by her children, her neighbors, her friends at church. They are all twittering about it behind her back, but no one is questioning whether it is a normal part of her aging, or whether there is some cause that can be fixed. A review of the medications she takes would show that she is taking one drug prescribed by her cardiologist, and another prescribed by her orthopedist, and those two drugs should never be taken together. But no one in the woman's life knows to do that review, nor do they know how to do that review.

- An elderly man has taken blood pressure meds for 10 years, always twice a day. But his doctor just changed the prescription to an 'extended release" drug, twice as potent, and necessary only once a day. The new instructions on the bottle are correct, but no one brought the difference to the man's attention and now he's taking twice as much of the drug - and will eventually get sicker or die from doing so.

Medical Errors Take a Toll on Quantity and Quality of Life for Patients and Their Families Too

It doesn't take rocket science to see the detrimental effects of medical errors and misdiagnosis. People get sicker, or they at least don't get well. Too many die.

There is nothing more abhorrent than preventable medical errors causing illness or death because the entire point of seeking medical care is to get well. Further, the negatives ripple in many directions. Sicker and more debilitated patients impact families and finances in terrible ways.

Patient Advocates - No Longer Just a Nicety

Having that objective, expert observer along for the journey can make an enormous difference when it comes to preventing medical errors. Here are some of the ways they can be life and quality-of-life saving:

- A patient advocate will help you find an objective second, third or fourth opinion knowing that doctors are friends, socialize outside of work, and therefore rarely contradict each other.

- A patient advocate will coordinate your care among your many doctors.

- A patient advocate won't be afraid to tell the next specialist that the last one already ordered your imaging or medical tests, saving you the hassle and the money new ones might cost.

- A patient advocate will ask the right questions on your behalf even when you have been scared into silence.

- A patient advocate will help you sort out a differential diagnosis. That's the process used to arrive at the right diagnosis.

- A patient advocate will sit by your bedside in the hospital making sure you are being taken care of properly. That means that she won't let anyone touch you unless their hands have been washed and sanitized, that you are being given the right drugs at the right times (even when you are sleeping), that when the call bell is pushed, someone actually shows up, and more.

- A patient advocate will help coordinate and oversee the transitions of care that usually present problems, including your return home from the hospital.

And many more.

Find direct links to the resources in this book at:

www.YouBetYourLifeBooks.com/10Reasons/Resources

Chapter Seven

Reason #6

The World Wide Web Is a Trap

Ahhh the Internet.

You may wonder, like I do, how you ever lived without it! We have instant information at our fingertips. We can learn everything we need to learn to help us understand our symptoms or even to diagnose ourselves.

In fact, we have access to too much, including websites for which "helping patients" isn't even a goal. They are the moneymakers. Their goal is about making money whether they are helpful to us or not.

I'm sure that doesn't surprise you. You may even be nodding your head. Of course they just want to make money! That's how the system works!

And you think because you are so very savvy to this fact, that it protects you from believing harmful information.

Unfortunately, for most of us, that's just not true. Here are five reasons why not:

1. At the point we rely on the web for our healthcare information, too many of us let our emotions get in the way of how and what we read. (Read more about the detriment of emotions in Reason #2: Emotions Can Get in Your Way) For some of us, that means we will hang on desperately to any shred of positive information, putting us in denial of reality. For others, that

means we'll glom on to the most negative of information, positive we have developed brain cancer or another dread disease, or that the care we are going to need will cost us our life savings.

2. Healthcare moneymakers know desperate people, or even hopeful people, will believe what they are told about this treatment, or that drug, or this surgery, or that medical device, simply because of that desperation.

3. Entire marketing departments of these money-makers exist simply to be there to capitalize on that desperation. The web, combined with TV advertising, are their two main vehicles for doing so because those tools take them inside the worried patient's or caregiver's home and head.

4. As the emotional patients we are, we find great relief in the information they provide us, and are rendered almost (please note - "almost") incapable of sorting out the truth from the fiction the moneymakers want us to believe.

5. On top of these reasons about emotions, we are - well - lazy! We do a web search, using key words or phrases, and we check out the top few results. Maybe we read all the references on the first page of search results - or maybe only a few.....

   What most of us don't realize is that many of those top results are simply (more!) advertisements. Further, we don't realize that the information we have found was built to find us, then fool us.

   There is specific coding called "meta data" built into webpages to make them show up at the top of search engines. Anyone who wants to sell you something knows how to do this coding, and it's one of the ways they can make sure you find their information; information that will help you - or fool you. As long as they make money, they don't care which.

Which Web Information is Most Problematic?

In varying degrees, any information that has been supplied by a healthcare moneymaker is at least suspect, if not downright dangerous. Remember - their goal is to make money whether or not they help you. Their information may look as if it's intended to help... and it is! It's intended to help them.

These problematic websites range widely in their ability to harm you. Examples:

♦ A pharmaceutical website presents a very slick and informative website about a disease you have been diagnosed with (or have self-diagnosed yourself with.) Citations of the drug they want you to buy are sprinkled throughout the site, usually with an "ask your doctor" command. By the time you've spent enough time on that site, you will be convinced to ask your doctor about it, and may eventually be prescribed it, even if there might have been another drug or treatment that would have been just as effective, more effective, and possibly less expensive for you.

♦ A knee or hip replacement manufacturer shows on its website healthy older people running and playing with their grandchildren - all smiles - as if they have no care in the world. They explain why THEIR knee or hip is THE knee or hip you need, and provide a list of doctors who use their devices. You choose one of those doctors, very sure that this is the right choice for you. Maybe it is, but maybe it isn't. The problem is, those doctors will rarely give you an objective opinion. It's akin to going to the Ford dealer for a used car, when in fact, the better car for you might be a Chevy. How many Ford dealers are going to sell you a Chevy?

♦ Your local hospital touts the great doctors on their staff. You see smiling and capable-looking physicians working with much-like-you patients. You feel some peace of mind they can do a good job for you, and you call to make an appointment. What you don't know is that the very doctor you've been assigned to has a malpractice track record, or has been cited and sanctioned for abusing his patients. [19]

♦ An alternative care clinic promises to cure you of the terminal cancer you have developed. They make grand promises on their website[20] and you - in your desperation - buy in.

Now - as you read this, probably fairly healthy and not yet in this stage of desperation - you probably think you would never fall for

---

19   Read the disturbing and scary story of Dr. Michael T. Clarke, who is still performing surgery every day. http://www.syracuse.com/health/index.ssf/2015/05syracuse_doc_accused_of_slapping_patients_fined_10000_ordered_to_get_therapy.html

20   http://www.camelotcancercare.com/

this type of sham. But I am aware of this clinic because I was contacted in 2006 by a man who was so desperate that he reached out to me to ask if I thought it was bona fide, and if I thought they could help him. They wanted $10,000 to get started with his workup - that didn't even include treatment. I told him I could not make a decision for him, but in a million years, I would not spend my children's inheritance to go there. He went anyway. He spent tens of thousands of dollars. Then he died a few months later.

How to Avoid Snake Oil, Mis- and Disinformation on the Web

So how are you supposed to know which references can really help you? Or which ones won't?

There are ways to figure out what information is objective, and what is not, based on following the money, and figuring out the motivation of the organization that has put the information online for you.

Patient Advocates Can Find the Objective, Useful, and Reliable Information You Need

The problem, of course, is that when you are sick, or overwhelmed, or experiencing any of the FUDGE emotions including anger - you just can't do that same objective exploration. It's just not possible. You would have to be superhuman.

However, patient advocates don't have the same constraints you do. Most patient advocates who provide healthcare system navigation services have the ability to dig up the information you can trust, and avoid the information you cannot. Further, there are advocates who do only this kind of research. In fact, they know how to dig deep into the hidden parts of the web to get information you might never find, including clinical trials, or malpractice, or even good options for medical tourism where you can go outside the country to get treatment at a much reduced price.

Chapter Eight

Reason #7

You're Not Making Your Own Decisions

If you are a typical patient, everyone else around you is making your healthcare-related decisions. The most important person, the person who should have the most say-so in deciding what your next steps should be, is constantly being overruled by others. That's you.

Consider these scenarios:

You see your doctor, you go for tests. You return to the doctor who says, "Mr. Jones, your test results tell us that you have Disease X. See? Here's this result, and here's that result. So this is how we treat Disease X...."

You, stunned, go along, taking the doctor's every word as gospel, following his recommendations like a lemming to the sea.

...or...

Two days after the explanation from the doctor, and after you've returned home to await the call from the nurse who will tell you where and when to be somewhere for treatment for Disease X, you instead receive a phone call telling you to return to the doctor's office. Your insurer won't give permission for the Disease X Treatment recommended by your doctor.

...or...

You stand up to the doctor and tell him, "Forget it! I don't want treatment! I'd rather just see what happens than put up with the side effects you've described!" Feeling so very in-control, you go home to tell your spouse about your decision... whereupon your spouse freaks. What do you MEAN you won't get treated? How will you go on with life? What will happen to the rest of the family if you DIE? Or Can't WORK? And so you relent, go back to see your doctor, and get on with the doctor's recommended treatment.

...or... switching gears away from your own medical situation....

You've been Dad's caregiver for several years now. He lives a few blocks away, and since Mom died, you've taken care of him while he stays in his home. You do all his shopping, you leave meals in his freezer (including specific instructions on how to warm them up), you clean his house, you take him to his doctor appointments, and every few Sundays you take him to church. Your teenager cuts his lawn, and your husband picks him up every Thursday to bring him to your house for dinner.

But now Dad is struggling, and you can no longer keep up with him, your kids, your husband, your home and of course, your job. It's time for Dad to move to a nursing home. You discuss it with Dad, and with your husband, too. They agree, and you begin to look into options.

Until your brother finds out. He lives 800 miles away, visits Dad once every two years, and calls Dad for two reasons - Christmas, and because he needs money, which Dad, of course, sends to him. During one of those calls, Dad mentions to your brother that you think Dad needs to move to a nursing home and brother goes ballistic. Brother calls you and tells you on no uncertain terms that Dad will NOT go into a nursing home because it will cost brother his inheritance to pay for nursing home care. You can't reason with your brother. He has always been a bully. And since that phone call, Dad is being less cooperative....

So - just who is making your decisions?

Granted, sometimes it is very difficult to make your own decisions, then follow through with them.

Your doctor doesn't want to get into a long conversation about options for all the time-constraint reasons cited in Reason #3. It's far easier, and usually more lucrative for them to just tell you what you should do, then see that you do it.

Your insurer doesn't want to pay for one bit of treatment more than they must, as required by contract or standard of care. But that doesn't mean they'll turn you down only for those things. They'll turn you down for anything they can get away with, whether or not they are, by contract, obligated to pay for it. Further, so few patients actually fight to get what they need or want that it works - it saves payers lots of money to turn down their patients for care the insurer doesn't want to pay for. If the patient fights for coverage later - well - OK. But why pay for it if they don't have to?

And then there are the people we love. Granted, we might want to take their wishes into account, but seriously - whose life is it? Why should you have to put up with one extra minute of pain or debilitation? For example, maybe you prefer not to suffer through chemo just to buy yourself an extra few months of life. Loved ones see our decisions through their own lenses and may miss the obvious signs of your struggle.

Decision by consensus is never easy when there are too many decision-makers involved, as seen in the illustration of the brother who stands in the way of Dad and the nursing home. Similar scenarios play themselves out every day. Families can be destroyed by hurt feelings over these difficult health-related decisions that must be made.

Making Your Own Decisions

The key is taking back ownership of your decision-making. When you are sick, debilitated, exhausted, scared, bullied and all those problematic emotions described in Reason #2, then it's almost impossible to do that on your own.

That's where a professional patient advocate comes in. The role he or she plays is a bit different for this particular reason. Here she will step in as a sounding board, one that can negotiate when need be.

A professional advocate can help you toot your decision horn. He can help you discuss options with your doctor. He can help you get coverage from your insurer for treatments the insurer may tell you won't be covered. He may help you discuss your needs for making certain choices with your family. And yes, he can help you stand up to your bullying brother.

To be clear - your patient advocate will never make a decision on your behalf. Your advocate's job is to be sure you have all the information you need - objective and thorough - to make decisions yourself. If others must get involved (like loved ones, whether or not the involvement is contentious), they can find someone to help you negotiate the right answers.

Among Your Most Important Decisions: Advance Directives

There is one more very important aspect to decision-making. That is; development of your advance directives.

Advance directives are those end-of-life decisions and documents we should all have at the ready for when they are needed. Wills, living wills, or DNRs (Do Not Resuscitate orders), POLST (Physician Orders for Life Sustaining Treatment) or MOLST (Medical Orders for Life Sustaining Treatment). Every state has different rules and expectations for your advance directives.

I hear frequently from people who wish their loved ones would be willing to discuss with them their end-of-life wishes. Sometimes they aren't even sure what their wishes are because they don't really understand their options. Others have specific wishes, but find their loved ones don't agree, and they have very little confidence their wishes will be carried out when the time comes.

Again - professional advocates to the rescue. These professionals know the ins and outs of advance directives. They know how to walk you through the conversation, and they know how to engage your loved ones in the conversation, too. They know what paperwork needs to be completed, and where it needs to be stored (like - NEVER in a safe deposit box!) They know if you need a lawyer or a notary. And they can be there at the moment your decisions need to be invoked, making sure your wishes are the ones being followed.

The peace of mind you'll feel with those decisions and paperwork behind you can be enormous.

Find direct links to the resources in this book at:

www.YouBetYourLifeBooks.com/10Reasons/Resources

Chapter Nine

Reason #8

You've Probably Got the Wrong Health Insurance Plan

When I suffered my misdiagnosis in 2004, I was self-employed, with self-employed person's health insurance.

My insurance was a high deductible plan. It had the lowest premium ($484 a month for one, non-smoking person - in 2004 dollars). I had a $5000 deductible (meaning, I had to pay out $5000 before insurance would kick in at all), and then it was a 60/40 split - for every $100 medical bill, they would pay $60 and I would pay $40.

In those days, pre-Affordable Care Act (Obamacare) it was the only insurance affordable for someone like me - or so I thought. I felt like I was lucky to have health insurance at all.

I hate to tell you this, but my "low priced, high-deductible" health insurance almost put me into bankruptcy. My misdiagnosis cost me every penny I had, except that I didn't lose my house and I didn't lose my retirement savings. It took me years to make up the differences. Truth is, I'm still working on it.

So why do I share all this?

Because like I did, you probably have the wrong health insurance plan, too.

But wait! (you say) I have Medicare! My healthcare is free!

Oh no - it's not! If you think that, then you are in for a rude awakening should you ever be faced with a real health challenge.

Thing is - I thought I was being smart. I thought that I would keep my premiums down, then if something really happened I would just pull the difference from my savings.

The problem is "the difference." I didn't really understand the differences.

Here are some examples - differences we don't think about:

- The plan you have also determines the doctors you can see, and the hospitals and testing labs you can go to. They are listed as to whom you are allowed to see. If they aren't on the list, you'll pay to see them out of your own pocket. This can become highly problematic in several ways (which we will examine more closely in Reason #9.)

- The plan you have determines your co-pay for both visits and treatments. A lower premium means higher co-pays. So even if you save $100 a month on the premium (with its restrictions on which doctors you can see) - you might make that up in two co-pays anyway - seeing doctors who aren't your first choice.

- Lower premium plans also put you on drug formularies with higher co-pays. So, for example, when you pick up your child's prescription for allergy medicine you might have to pay $30 for the drug each month on the lower premium insurance, but only $5 a month for the same drug on the higher premium insurance. In the span of a year, that's a $300 difference - more from your pocket. And that's only one prescription.

- Now let's talk hospitals... the lower premium insurance plans tend to allow admissions at the worst rated hospitals. Now - that's a generalization - and it won't always be true. But it's most definitely something you need to look at when you are choosing your insurance plan.

- The bottom line is that sometimes the seemingly "best deal" in health insurance, just isn't that at all.

Choosing the Right Plan for You

So how can you tell which is the right plan for you?

The right plan will consist of one that lets you see the doctors you want to see, at the facilities you want to see them in, as frequently as you need to see them. It will allow you to be tested in the ways you and your doctor think you need to be tested, and it will let you be admitted to the hospital you believe is safest, and best. All that - at a price you are willing to pay.

I wish I could give you a formula for choosing this "right" health insurance plan. That would make it so much easier, wouldn't it? There are some out there, but they aren't easy to use, and the entire reason you're reading this book is because you already know you need some help.

Of course, our choices of health plans are usually quite limited. If you have an employer-sponsored plan, there may be only one choice, in which case - I do hope it works out for you.

If you have more than one choice, how are you supposed to choose the right one?

Well, that requires you to pull out your crystal ball...

...or contact your patient advocate.

Yes - this is one of the ways a patient advocate can pay for him or herself in actual money when hired. In probably no more than an hour, by making some educated guesses and assumptions using one of those magic formulas I mentioned above, you can work with a knowledgeable patient advocate to figure out which plan is the right one for you.

And then, do it again next year. You'll see why in our next reason....

Chapter Ten

Reason #9

Your Insurance Coverage
Is a Moving Target

One of the biggest mistakes we make regarding health insurance is thinking that once we've chosen a plan, it will be the right plan for next year, and the next, and the next....

Foolish! Truly foolish.

Plans change all the time. The doctors who subscribe to them change. Their coverages change. Their pricing changes. The facilities that will accept them change. Their rules for getting coverage changes...

All the time.

They don't want you to know that! They won't alert you. And the changes don't always take place in sync with when we make our plan choices.

- The doctor you saw last month may no longer be approved by your insurer. In fact, her practice is no longer accepting patients who have your insurance.

- You went to the ER in January when your temperature spiked over 103° but this month, when you slice open your knee, you'll need permission from your insurer before you go; otherwise you'll have to pay cash for the visit.

• If your elderly parent suffers a stroke and is taken to the ER, she may be put on "observation status" for a few days instead of being admitted to the hospital. Why? Because Medicare doesn't pay for patients who are on observation status, and if somehow the hospital thinks your mother can afford it (meaning - she has a credit card) they will just keep her overnight for a few nights, then send her a bill for $10,000 or more. She will have no recourse but to pay it.

• Your friend might need gall bladder surgery and knowing that, she took care of all the preparation ahead of time. She double checked that her surgeon was covered, that her hospital stay is covered, that all her drugs are covered... only to receive a bill a few months after discharge for the anesthesiologist who wasn't covered, and considered out-of-network.[21] Seriously.

Yes - your health insurance and its benefits to you are a moving target.

My most recent brush was when I needed blood work, a visit I make every six months prior to a checkup with my primary care doctor. I've always gone to a lab just a mile from my home, 8 am, in and out (because I want breakfast and can't eat until after they draw that blood!) This time, knowing that insurance is a moving target, I called my insurer. I told them I was just double checking my coverage for the lab and sure enough - that lab is no longer working with my insurer. I had to go to a different one - this one more like a half-hour away. But, at least I didn't get caught in the "out of pocket" tangled web! No surprise for me, but I'm sure many others were surprised when they got bills for their lab work.

Here's the problem: your doctor doesn't know who or what is covered by your insurance. Your doctor is just telling you to get a test, or to fill a prescription, without regard to the cost, or how it will be paid. Even if you ask your doctor what lab to go to, or where the best pricing is for your prescription, your doctor will have no idea. It's just not information they maintain. Their patients are covered by hundreds, maybe thousands of different

---

21 In some states, the rules are changing for out-of-network coverage that results from these kinds of scenarios. In New York, it's called the "Surprise Bill" - meaning, patients should not be responsible for those surprises. http://consumersunion.org/surprise-medical-bills/

health plans. They only know which ones they work with, and how much they will be paid for each service on that plan. Period.

Since you are reading this book, there is a good chance you or a loved one has a health challenge that requires plenty of doctor visits, testing and treatment. Unless you have someone to track your insurance against those needs, you will get caught in that web, too.

So what are you supposed to do?

There are two ways a patient advocate can help you corral that moving target.

- First, they can try to help you prevent getting caught in an uncovered situation by double checking coverage prior to your access. They can stay in touch with your insurance people to make sure you are receiving only care that will be paid for. It's a headache! But it's a headache they know how to juggle on your behalf.

- Second, should you have already run into problems, and you're getting bills you didn't expect, they can negotiate with your insurer and possibly get them paid, or at least lowered.

Lowered - now there's a concept! We'll tackle that further in Reason #10, because yes, your medical bills are probably wrong.

Chapter Eleven

Reason #10

Your Medical Bills Are Probably Wrong

Picture this: You need surgery - maybe your gall bladder needs to be removed. You make sure all the paperwork is taken care of ahead of time, the insurance T's are crossed and I's are dotted.

You stay in the hospital for two days. Everything seems to go smoothly. You catch up on a couple of TV soap operas, read a book, chat with your roommate, and finally it's time to go home. Granted, there are some hassles through the discharge process (See Reason #5) - but your spouse gets you home, comfortable... and you convalesce exactly as you should.

Piece of cake.

Until... six weeks later a bill from the hospital arrives in the mail. $22,000 WHAAAT?

Clearly, there is something wrong!

The $75 box of tissues. The $300 massage the nurse offered you, but never mentioned you would pay extra for! The two CT scans you never had = $2500. A $40 a day charge for the TV. And a $1200 line item for a doctor who was brought in on a "consult." What doctor? Consulting about what?

You've recovered from your surgery, but how will you ever recover from this sort of bill? You don't even know how to read it or make sense of it. What are all those codes on it? And why on earth didn't your insurance pay for it? You were only there two days!

If you think this is at all unusual, think again. In fact, statistics tell us that up to 80% of hospital bills have mistakes.[22] Billing for the wrong thing, billing double for some things, billing for things that didn't even happen, billing for things you didn't know were extra - and more.

The average Jane or Joe doesn't have a clue how to get them sorted out and cleaned up. Further, even if they try, they will run into hospital brick walls. The hospital billing department not only doesn't care what happened to you while you were there, they don't care about getting your bill right. In fact, if they charge you too much, and you pay it, they are only rewarded for doing so.[23]

Some of the charges are probably fair, even if they don't seem that way. But others are totally unfair, and may be the result of balance billing, upcoding or unbundling, all of which may be illegal.

And you probably don't even know what balance billing, upcoding or unbundling mean. So how on earth will you be able to sort that bill out?

And - you have insurance. What about the people who don't have insurance, or don't have hospital coverage? For the hospital stay you had, with no insurance coverage, their bill could be more like $50,000. For the exact same services, an insurer would be expected to pay, maybe $7000.

What's wrong with this picture? Plenty.

The problem is - we aren't going to be the ones to fix this crazy system. And if you are the one who gets that bill, insurance or no, you need to get it cleared up - and paid - sooner, not later, before it is reflected on your credit score.

---

22 http://www.wsj.com/articles/
SB10001424052748703312904576146371931841968

23 It has been alleged that some hospitals reward their billing departments for padding bills when those bills get paid. I have never been able to corroborate that, but it would not surprise me.

Enter medical billing advocates - who can whip a hospital bill like yours into shape and - possibly - negotiate it to something that is far more manageable to you. Maybe even eliminate it all together.

These financial miracle workers have a variety of tools at their disposal - tools you cannot get your hands on, and don't even know to ask about. They have access to "chargemasters" - the hospital's list of charges for every service and product they offer and sell. They have access to code lists - CPTs, DRGs and others - that explain what the bill is supposed to cover. They know the terminology used to hide that $75 box of tissues. And they know the people at the hospital with whom they can negotiate.

Yes. You need a patient advocate.

Chapter Twelve

Find the Right Advocate: (Relax, You're in Good Hands)

Hopefully I've convinced you that you need a patient advocate in your corner. If I haven't, then reread some of those reasons.

You wouldn't go to jail without calling a lawyer to bail you out. And you shouldn't go into healthcare without a patient advocate by your side!

Now the key is to find the best patient advocate for you. You want someone who has the skills you need, with a fit for your personality, in a location that makes sense for you.

Where to Find a Patient Advocate

You might start by asking others if they have ever hired a private advocate, and if so, do they recommend the person they worked with?

You may also look in one of the online advocate directories. As of mid-2015, there are two.[24]

• **www.AdvoConnection.com** - The AdvoConnection Directory lists advocates throughout the US and Canada, by their location and the services they provide. It includes advocates who provide a range of services, from medical-navigational

---

24 We should note there is a great deal of crossover between these two directories. Most advocates are found in both directories. We should further note that as of mid-2015, there are no more than 250 private, professional patient advocates currently working with patients. If you live in a larger city or population area, you'll probably find advocates to help you, but you may struggle if you live in a less populated area.

advocacy, geriatric care, mediation, and insurance, medical billing and claims advocacy, too.

- **www.NAHAC.com** - The National Association for Health Advocacy Consultants directory contains advocates all over the US. Few, if any, are medical billing and claims advocates.

You can also do a general web search. Search for "patient advocate" and the state and/or city you live in. If you need help only with medical billing issues, you won't need to be so concerned with an advocate's location since that work can all be done virtually. You may never need to meet in person.

How to Choose the Right Advocate

There are a number of questions you'll want to ask a potential advocate before you hire him or her. Some of them relate to the advocate's qualifications. Others are focused on how your working relationship will be established.

A few things to know:

Private advocacy as a profession is quite new. There is not - yet - any sort of certification required for patient advocates[25], nor is there any specific type of education required. There are more than three dozen colleges, universities and organizations that offer some sort of educational program for people who want to become advocates, but there is no requirement to study any of them.

That means that the advocates you might choose from will need to be qualified in other ways. Thus, these questions are intended to pull the information from them that will help you qualify them.

Find one or more advocates online, perhaps in one of the directories, then call or phone. Make appointments to interview them. Provide a brief overview of your situation, then ask the following:[26]

- Have you handled other cases similar to mine?
  How long have you been a private, independent advocate?

- What are your credentials? Do you have background, training

---

25 http://aphablog.com/2011/01/03/the-myth-of-patient-advocacy-certification

26 These questions can also be found here: http://advoconnection.com/hire-a-patient-advocate/#interview

When you interview your potential advocate, be sure to ask how they arrive at a price, and what their terms are. Expect to pay up front for all or part of the work.

The Work Process

So what can you expect in your working relationship?

It would be rare for two advocate relationships to go exactly the same way. Every patient is different, every advocate is different, and every situation is different, of course.

But there are some basics to all patient advocacy processes, outlined here:

- **Step One:**
  Identify one or more advocates, interview them, and choose the one you would like to work with.

- **Step Two:**
  Your chosen advocate will provide you with a contract which will outline the working relationship, including the services to be provided, the scope of work, what it will cost, the payment terms, and how each of you can get out of the contract if you choose to.

- **Step Three:**
  You will make your first payment to your advocate.

- **Step Four:**
  The advocate will may ask for your signature on a HIPAA privacy form, and will then be able to acquire the medical records and/or bills necessary for the work.

- **Step Five:**
  You and your advocate will work together to complete the scope of work you have defined in your agreement. This may begin with an assessment which, once completed, means you go back through these steps again.

Depending on your situation and decisions along the way, your contract and scope of work may be amended to adjust to anything new that comes along.

After You and Your Advocate Work Together

I often hear from advocates that they develop close working relationships with their clients (yes, once you are under contract, you become the advocate's "client"). You and your advocate may stay in touch for months or years even when your work is done.

If your advocate is a good business person, and the relationship and work have gone well, she will ask you for a testimonial which she can use in her marketing. She may also ask you if you would like to share your story and journey with the media, should the media seek someone who fits your profile. Feel free to agree - or not - to any of these requests.

If you would like to write a testimonial to help your advocate, you can do so at the AdvoConnection Directory:

http://advoconnection.com/submit-a-testimonial-for-your-advocate/

Resources

Find direct links to the resources in this book at:

www.YouBetYourLifeBooks.com/10Reasons/Resources

We hope we've convinced you that hiring a private, professional patient advocate is not only in your best interest, but will provide you with the peace of mind you need as you weather the upcoming healthcare system storms that await you.

Whether you need an advocate for yourself, or for a loved one, or even for a good employee or member of your organization, we hope you have found this overview to be helpful.

Here are some additional resources to use as you move forward:

Directories of Patient Advocates

- www.AdvoConnection.com

- www.NAHAC.com

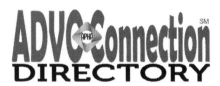

Articles

- What Services Do Patient Advocates Offer?
  http://patients.about.com/od/caringforotherpatients/a/advocatesvs.htm

- How to Interview and Choose a Patient Advocate
  http://patients.about.com/od/caringforotherpatients/tp/Choose-a-Patient-Advocate.htm

- Patient Advocates and Navigators, and the Allegiance Factor
  http://patients.about.com/od/caringforotherpatients/a/Allegiance-Factor-Can-A-Patient-Advocate-Or-Patient-Navigator-Help-You.htm

- Are Patient Advocates Certified or Credentialed?
  http://patients.about.com/od/caringforotherpatients/f/Are-Patient-Advocates-Certified-Or-Credentialed.htm

Book

You Bet Your Life! The 10 Mistakes Every Patient Makes (How to Fix Them to Get the Healthcare You Deserve)

http://youbetyourlifebooks.com/ purchase.htm

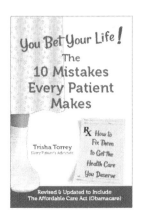

If you are interested in becoming a professional advocate yourself:

www.HealthAdvocateResources.com and

www.APHAdvocates.org

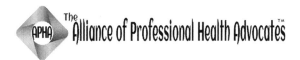

The Health Advocate's code of Conduct and Professional Standards

1. Health advocates practice with compassion and respect for the patients, clients and families with whom they work.

2. Health advocates' primary commitments are to promote the health, safety, and rights of their patients and clients.

3. Health advocates will, at all times, be transparent in their work with clients. They will disclose to clients their credentials, experience, pricing structure, and any financial relationships they hold with other professionals, businesses or institutions.

4. Health advocates will, at all times, maintain privacy on behalf of their patients and clients and will keep confidential all activities and records according to agreements among them, and any applicable laws.

5. Health advocates will guide and assist their clients-patients in medical decision-making but at no time will make decisions about health or medical care or payment for medical services on their behalf.

6. Health advocates will promote use of their client-patients' values and belief systems as the foundation for their decision-making.

7. Health advocates will, at all times, practice within their competency. Any requests for services outside the advocate's expertise will be referred to someone else who is equipped to provide those services to ensure the client-patient is benefitting from the best knowledge base.

8. Health advocates will, at all times, work within their professional boundaries and will reject any requests or demands that would cause them to violate those boundaries. Such violations may include, but not be limited to, accepting money or gifts as compensation for referrals to other professionals, fulfilling requests to perform illegal or unethical actions, agreeing to provide services outside any geographical limits, developing a romantic or sexual relationship with a client or someone related to the client, agreeing to perform any duties without the disclosure or input needed from the client, or any other circumstances that could result in conflicts-of-interest or the inability to fully perform the work the two parties have agreed upon.

9. Health advocates will not discriminate. They will at no time refuse to work with someone due to that person's race, religion, culture, gender, or sexual preference.

10. Health advocates will continue to pursue education to further their knowledge base, skill set, and practice in order to provide client-patients with the most current information relevant to his/her health situation.

Find this code at: http://HealthAdvocateCode.org

About the Author

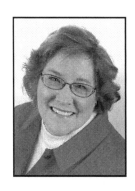

When Trisha Torrey was diagnosed with a rare, aggressive and terminal form of lymphoma in 2004, she was a web marketing consultant who knew little or nothing about getting decent medical care. She was naïve to the dysfunction of the American healthcare system that was tasked with treating her.

Initially Trisha made every mistake a patient could make. But she got smart, fast. She learned that the possibility of excellent care was too easily and frequently eclipsed by profit-motives, miscommunication and mistakes. She also learned that if she didn't stick up for herself, and insist on the help she needed, she would not get it.

Once Trisha put that cancer odyssey behind her, she decided it was up to her to sound the warning bells about the dysfunction, and apply her skills to teaching others how to navigate the dangerous landscape of American healthcare. She sold her marketing company in 2006 to devote herself full time to the cause.

Today Trisha calls herself "Every Patient's Advocate." She writes and speaks on topics of interest to patients, patient advocates and medical professionals. This is her sixth book.

She also founded and is director of the Alliance of Professional Health Advocates, the group of professionals found in the AdvoConnection Patient Advocate Directory.

She has been quoted by or appeared on CNN, MSNBC, NPR, the *Wall Street Journal, U.S. News and World Report*, Fox, *Forbes, O Magazine, Health Magazine*, and others.

Trisha lives in Central New York State with her husband, Butch, and her mini-mutt, Crosby. When she's not doing her patient advocacy thing, she enjoys playing golf, gardening, working in stained glass, travel and spending time in the Adirondack Mountains.

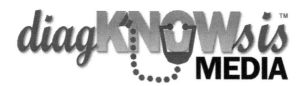

More from DiagKNOWsis Media

The DiagKNOWsis family of patient-centered media.

www.DiagKNOWsis.com

www.EveryPatientsAdvocate.com

www.AdvoConnection.com

www.APHAdvocates.org

www.HealthAdvocateResources.com

www.YouBetYourLifeBooks.com

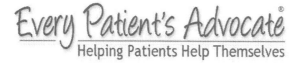

Helping Patients Help Themselves

Made in the USA
Lexington, KY
03 February 2019